Where the Sun Don't Shine

Surviving Colon Cancer

with Humor, Hope and Support

Where the Sun Don't Shine

Surviving Colon Cancer
with Humor, Hope and Support

Barry "Jack" Frost

Bell Bottom
Press

Copyright © 2021 by Barry Frost

All rights reserved. Printed in the United States of America. No part of this book may be reproduced or used in any manner whatsoever without the express written permission of the publisher except for the use of brief quotations in a book review.

ISBN 978-0-578-79273-6

Bell Bottom Press
Loveland, Colorado

Cover design by Robin Locke Monda

For Laraine

CONTENTS

Cancer?	15
Hope Is Ever Present	19
Operation Removal	26
Visions	31
On the Third Day	36
Karma Buster	41
Recovery Time	43
Back to Work	49
Break Down	53
A Voice Out of the Blue	55
The Support Group	61
Turnovers with Sadness and Joy	68
Saying Goodbyes	72
Tea and Crumpets Anyone	74
Staying the Course	79
All Work and No Play	83
My New Pet	86
The First End Game and Then	90
Getting Radical	93

CONTENTS, continued

Facing the Support Group	99
Departing is Such Sweet Sorrow	102
Letting Go and a Close Call	195
Moving Day	110
Help is on the Way	114
Life is Good	116
Advice for Cancer Patients and Care Givers	119

ACKNOWLEDGMENTS

The person I would most like to acknowledge here is my strong and steadfast wife, Laraine. Laraine stood by me one hundred per cent throughout my whole cancer ordeal. I was sad, happy, worried, exhausted, frail, or strong, depending on the day, but this didn't deter Laraine from having my back at all times. This made a tremendous difference to the whole movie. Yes, it often seemed like I was acting in a movie about life, loyalty, and love.

A special mention must go to the two nurses that came to Laraine and my bedside in the recovery room after my colonoscopy. Their kindness and loving spirit helped calm us down as we were told I had cancer.

For me, McKee Hospital Cancer Center has to be the greatest cancer center on the planet. The people there showed love and kindness, as well as dedication to not only their job but to the individual patient. Their unbridled thoughtfulness was and is exemplary.

There are too many individuals and small groups to praise and thank individually, so please forgive me for lumping you all together. My many supporters included friends, family, individual testing labs, the electrical company I worked for (Precision Service Electric), doctors and nurses, and even the cleaning staff of all those facilities. Thank you all so very much for all your good deeds, kindness, and loving support. I could not have made the journey without you.

Finally I am so very grateful to have been introduced to my editor, Cheryl Miller Thurston. She has been my rock for getting this book published. There is so much I don't know in this area, but Cheryl has guided me through the thicket of knowledge without complaint. This guidance has meant so much to me.

Thanks to you all again, including any I may have overlooked.

Barry "Jack'"Frost

INTRODUCTION

It is important for me to let you know that this book is not intended to guide anybody through the trauma of cancer. Many years ago I personally fought the good fight for two and a half years and lived to tell this tale.

There is no magic bullet or particular way to stay positive and hold one's head above water. I say this because everybody is different, subtly or dramatically. There are multiple levels of attitude, both good and bad. There are different reactions by everybody to the same chemo, and there are many, many, different kinds of chemo. The body's reaction to radiation is different and also depends on the strength and number of treatments administered. The financial state of people is different and can cause more stress (Cancer feeds on stress.) Some people have insurance and some don't. Some lose their job and therefore their insurance. Some can use religious or spiritual support, others not so much. There are those with the support of great family and/or friends, while others are more lonely. The list goes on and on.

It is so important to remember that people with the exact same type and stage of cancer can and will have totally different experiences, both inwardly and outwardly.

In this book I try to give a sense of how I handled my own unique set of circumstances. I will carry you through how and when I discovered the cancer, how I handled it, and how I survived mentally and physically. If you are a cancer patient, maybe it can help you. My hope is that it might give you a rough pathway to acknowledge and mold for your own needs.

Do try and allow some humor into your life, try to stay as positive as possible, and try to stay the course. I wish you good luck for your journey and a recovery that is as swift as possible. It can take a lot of work but you are worth it, don't ever forget that.

Barry

CANCER?

It was April 1. Yes, April Fools' Day—the day I discovered I had cancer. Probably not many people in the world would pick that particular day for such a monumental, life changing discovery, but I managed it with ease.

What? What? The news was a dagger in the heart and brain, thrust by an uncaring blank-faced doctor with no emotion or tact.

Several days earlier in the bathroom at night, I'd had a sensation of something hitting the floor between my feet. I turned the light on to find a glob of blood splatted on the rug. After cleaning it up, I retreated to bed and slept like a log.

The next day I phoned my GP for an appointment. When I met with him two days later, his immediate call was for me to have a colonoscopy as soon as possible. He said he would diagnose the situation once more information was available. I was thinking a bad case of hemorrhoids, but I now know what he suspected and probably knew for sure. I respect him greatly for not jumping to any conclusions on such a devastating subject. Two days later, after drinking fourteen gallons of goop, or so it seemed, I lay prostrate and vulnerable on a metal table in a fetal position. That camera is going where? I thought to myself as the smiling attendees went about their business, seeming so relaxed and normal. "It's going to be okay," they said. "You won't feel a thing. Just relax."

That's what you think on the other end of the lens, I thought. *Easy for you to say.*

They administered a shot into the tube they had punctured my wrist with, and then a nurse walked into the room. As she prepared to wheel me out of the room with all the colonoscopy equipment, I asked her what she was doing. She replied that she was taking me to the recovery room. At this, I politely told her I had not been scoped yet, to which she said, "Yes, you have." After some back and forth on the argument, she won the day. This was mainly because I was still partially in la-la land, and she held the high ground with me helpless on a moving platform.

The two nurses in the recovery room told me that most people go through thinking that nothing has happened yet because the drug they administer gives patients short term memory loss. Having seen the size of that camera I thought it just as well.

My wife Laraine was waiting for me, sitting on a chair next to where I ended up. Ha, ended up. Hmmmm.

She held my hand and smiled, waiting for me to be more coherent. The door of the room swung half open, and the doctor's head flopped around the leading edge. "You have cancer," he said, and the head disappeared forever. I never saw him again, which was just as well. His name was Pipe, which I thought appropriate for doing colonoscopies. What a jerk.

The two nurses, who were across the room a ways, looked at each other, and their jaws dropped. They both made haste to my bedside and felt awful for what had just happened. Their love and caring was very evident throughout their whole beings, and their apologies were profuse and sincere. Through my now tear-filled eyes, I assured them it wasn't their fault. Laraine and I hugged and clutched each other, oh, so very tightly.

This was the beginning of one of my biggest life lessons: It is okay to cry wherever, whenever, and for as long as you like. Let it all flood out and relieve the pressure, just like opening up a valve in the Hoover Dam. Believe me, within moments, the stress level is alleviated even if for just a short time. You can always do it again and again. I have cried with friends, I have cried by myself, I have cried while giving a talk on stage to hundreds of people. It just doesn't matter.

A while later and when I was somewhat more composed, we were ushered out by the discharge associate, having being given instructions to attend the hospital cancer center. The cancer center was attached to the hospital but around the other side and kind of tacked on the end. Rather like a tumor, I suppose. We eventually found it and entered through the two sets of sliding, automatic doors. I thought it strange that a man was standing outside attached to a metal stand with a tube going into him, presumably with chemo drugs, while smoking a cigarette. I wondered if he had to cough up the money for the treatment. Yeah, I know, that was bad, but I couldn't help it.

The staff at the reception desk knew that I was a new patient because they recognized all of their existing patients' names and faces. I soon learned that these people had the right balance of empathy while staying professional and stalwart. They were the epitome of excellence, love and understanding.

HOPE IS EVER PRESENT

A woman in a long, flowing white coat invited us to her lair, and the process of my treatment for the next two and a half years began. She was the doctor of all wonderful doctors.

She went over multiple scenarios with us and explained a kind of planning route for us to follow until everybody knew more about the situation and how bad it was. "Don't panic, at least not yet," was the message. At this point in the journey my eyes were still a little glazed, and although I was trying to listen with intent, it was difficult. Multiple live, color images were whipping through my mind as if a fast moving old film was rushing across a projector's lens.

My future was before me as a black curtain, and I was unable to see tomorrow with any clarity. It's strange because at the same time a second part of my mind was somewhat relaxed and seeing my world beyond the cure. How could both bleakness and hope occupy the same space at the same time? But did it matter? Any time spent worrying about trivial nonsense took away from concentrating upon my predicament and recovery.

We were then introduced to a radiologist who was also very kind. I had some x-rays taken of my abdomen from every angle around the sun, including where the sun don't shine, and we departed.

On the way home, we stopped at the office of my work place to relay the news to my boss. I was an electrician, and it is a job that requires strength and drive to make any money in the profession. How would he react? I needed the insurance, among other things, to be able to fight this good fight with all the tools available at once.

The first thing he said to us was, "Don't worry. You will always have a job here." John gave me great comfort that day and showed all the hallmarks of a good man and boss.

As we pulled into the garage at home, tears were beginning to creep through my eyeballs again, along with Laraine's. We both sat in silence holding hands, still in the garage, not knowing how to say the right thing, not knowing how to feel.

My spiritual path has involved me in a worldwide religious movement called Eckankar, which teaches a word to use to connect with God and spirit. The word is "HU" and is the Sanskrit name for God. I like to think that is why we are called human beings: man of HU, man of God, human. Just a personal thought process that makes sense to me. Laraine and I sang or chanted "HU" in a long drawn out fashion for quite a while. It helped us connect with God and calmed and relaxed us. We did not ask for help, as in prayer, but just let it be and trusted in any guidance that might be given. We were both extremely quiet for the rest of the evening and waited for the trip back to the radiologist the next day.

The radiologist was a somewhat strange sort of man whom we liked right from the outset. On entering his conference room, he dimmed the lights to show us on the wall the glowing images from the previous day. He had a pointer stick and prodded it at the image of my lower large intestine while saying, "This is shit," in a very matter of fact way. Laraine and I just about lost it as he continued unabashed after his last statement. We were snickering for quite a while as we tried to compose ourselves.

He continued explaining the slides and pointed out the cancer that was very close to the rectum. This concerned him, but I am sure he wasn't letting us know how much.

We now had to wait for a couple of days until a board of oncologists convened, which they did once a week, to discuss all new and ongoing cases and their progress. Then we were called into the cancer center and sat before the oncologist. She told me she was going to need a sample of the mass to be taken from my orifice, and I was to meet a surgeon in yet another area of the hospital.

Soon after, I once again lay prone and helpless, in fear of what was going to happen next. In the sterile room on the sterile table, my butt was bared for all to attack. This time, attack they did. With no drugs administered, some surgical scissors were eased into the darkness, and excruciating pain seared through my passageway. I had not seen an open fire to this point, so I wondered where they had got the red hot coals to sear the inside of my intestines.

Now I was, or used to be anyway, a rugby player. The word pain generally means nothing to us roughy-toughy men who play. However, this intrusion into my posterior was more than I wanted to handle. The apologies of the surgeon didn't do anything for the clenching of my teeth and stifled screams fighting to escape from my larynx. The doctor took three chunks of my cancerous flesh by cutting with what seemed like rose pruning shears.

The ordeal over, I was left to return my frazzled, crying body to normal. Normal was a word that had now shifted to another position in my new world.

It was at this juncture that I remembered what was said to me by my general practitioner at the very beginning of this journey. "Y'know," he said looking over the top of his glasses in a schoolteacher type manner, "A colonoscopy six months ago could have saved you a whole lot of trouble." Now he wasn't being a know-it-all or a Monday morning quarterback. He and I had a great relationship and wonderful rapport. We always swapped a joke between us during a visit. I would chide him about being a wussy soccer player and he reminded me of how crazy I was to play rugby. He was just pointing out the truth of the matter.

Right now and right here I am going to implore everybody to get a colonoscopy before the age of fifty—yes, before the age of fifty. The earlier the better. I had no family history of cancer of any kind and was as fit as a fiddle. My eating habits, while not perfect, were very good and nutritional.

You actually do not feel anything at all with a colonoscopy. It is a painless outpatient procedure, quick and simple and so beneficial. If there is any sign of cancer or pre-cancer, it can be dealt with instantly. Before you reach the end of this book (Why do I keep writing *end?)* go and do it. Do not procrastinate, do not hesitate, and do not pass go. You could be saving yourself a whole lot of trouble.

Go on, just go. What are you waiting for?

Again, the waiting for results. Waiting was the new game in town. I had to adjust my mind to this wait-and-see, cat-and-mouse scenario that would be with me for quite a while.

On returning to the room of torture, Laraine and I waited for the surgeon to come in. A nurse handed us a pamphlet that described four types of operation that could be performed, depending on the actual location of the cancer. I remember saying, "The first three types don't sound so bad, but the fourth one is definitely out. I'm not going to do that." The fourth choice involved removing the whole rectum and being given another avenue to excrete from. They called it a *colostomy*, a word I wasn't familiar with, for sure.

In came Doctor Death. You guessed it. The only real option, as it turned out, was option number four: removing the rectum and living with a colostomy for the rest of my life. If I didn't choose that option now, I would still have to go through it in a year or two. The odds of the cancer returning were almost one hundred percent without the colostomy. The nodes were too close to the sunlight to be able to remove all the cancer without the loss of said door to the outside world.

Devastation, more fear, and tears ensued. Was this a nightmare or was I really doing this? I started to think of people with cancer who had suffered on a long term basis. Surely my demise would be short lived at least? I begrudgingly signed the required paperwork to agree with this demolition of my body's nether regions. The fight was on. Let the battles commence; I had a war to win.

More meetings ensued with the oncologist and radiologist. After much study of my images by the whole cancer team, the radiation team went to work. The first move was to give me four tattoos. I thought of a popular tattoo when I was in the Royal Navy—a full blown fox hunt with the fox disappearing into his den. (Imagine where that ends up.) It was a very large tattoo, and not all men were gutsy enough to endure all that pain.

I didn't get a choice of tattoos, though. Four small crosses were indelibly inked into my skin. I have them even now, nineteen years later. This was done so that the radiation machine could line up exactly in the same place all forty-six times I was to be cooked. With the tattoos, the targeted area could be smaller, and the full weight of the treatment would come to bear exactly on the offending cancer cells every time. My torso endured another session of baring all my parts to the staff. I had often said, "Bottoms up!" in a pub before ordering a round of drinks, but this was different.

On another occasion I was asked, within a specific area of the belly, exactly where I would like the opening for the colostomy; it's called the stoma. For that placement, which they marked with an indelible ink pen, I brought along my electrician's tool belt. I put it on, and they marked the best spot where the belt would not be pressing on said *stoma*, or opening. I planned to continue working, no matter what. This was a must for my state of mind and, as it turned out, my cure.

OPERATION REMOVAL

The day of the races was upon us. I say us because Laraine and I were in this together, forming a two-pronged attack from different angles. Laraine's support and steadfastness was crucial to my survival, no ifs ands or butts. (Humor was going to become an integral and important part of my eventual support system. I couldn't resist that one could I?)

I have to interject here that I had now made dozens of phone calls to friends and immediate family members. At the beginning of each phone call, I broke down, unable to complete the opening sentences for several seconds. Laraine offered to make these calls, but I insisted it was something I needed to do. The strange thing is that, once the initial contact had been made and my situation discussed, subsequent calls were perfectly normal as far as emotions were concerned.

When I told somebody face to face that I had cancer, their eyes and body language told me a story. They wanted, so desperately, to ask me how long I had, but it felt too awkward for them. Let's face it; it's a heck of a statement to make. So with my inner voice I would say, "I'm going to outlive you, you son of a gun." This was a game for myself and brought a moment of fun and joy to me. I know, it's weird, but it helped me along the road, and every step is vital.

Anyway, I digress. The surgeon had re-established contact with me in the operation prep area and was making sure I understood what was about to take place. I'm guessing he didn't want me waking up to parts of my body missing without me being fully aware of it beforehand.

I did tell him that, if it was at all possible, he was to save my aperture, even if I had only a remote chance of success. He assured me he would do his best. My veins had already been prepped for the anesthesiologist, and I was going only partially into the land of nod at first. They needed my cooperation in the operation room before going fully under. My instructions were to play my CD of the HU song during the procedure, but if the surgeons started nodding off they could stop the chant.

While they were prepping themselves, and me, I told them one of my jokes. Since the surgeon was of German descent, I asked if he knew why the streets of Paris were lined with trees. Of course, he didn't know. The answer was "because Germans like to march in the shade."

The whole room burst out laughing as the loosey-goosey juice began coursing through my blood vessels. The room disappeared, and the next thing I knew I was being wheeled down a hall way and into a hospital room. I could barely see and could only just murmur some words in a very low voice. I saw Laraine and quietly said, "Who is this woman? She has been following me around for days. Call the cops." I remember people chuckling and Laraine saying, "He's going to be okay. He still has his sense of humor."

I was somewhat unceremoniously tipped into my new bed, and then I mapped out the back of my eyelids for quite a while. When I eventually came to, a kind, warm hand was holding mine. As I became conscious and at least a little aware, I felt below the sheets, hoping to find my whole body intact.

It wasn't.

Everything that could sink sank. I couldn't speak, but tears rolled down my cheeks as the curtain was being raised on my new life. Why? Why? Why? There was nothing my loving wife could do or say. She was as sad as I was and teared up with me while squeezing my hand a little tighter.

After a while, the surgeon came in and was so nice to us both. Even though he had done this procedure hundreds of times, he made it seem as if I was his first patient. He was caring and empathetic. He told me that while in there, y'know, "in there," he was right next to my appendix. He asked if it was okay that he took it out. "You have no need for it anyway, and it could save you possible trouble in the future."

I told him, "No. You need to put it back." Even in one of my darkest hours I could still mess with the best. We all had a little chuckle, and I thanked him for being so diligent and progressive.

The piece of not so good news the surgeon also brought was that I had stage four cancer, not stage three as at first thought. He had taken fourteen lymph nodes from the site, and eleven of them had cancer. This meant the cancer could now go willy-nilly through my body via the lymph system.

The darker it got, the lighter I had to become.

He left us, promising to check on me later in the day. The very attentive staff asked what my pain level was, and I told them I was not in any pain. They told me I would be and to let them know as soon as I was not comfortable. It is easier for a patient to head off pain at the pass than to try to remove pain afterwards. I told them that I understood their philosophy, and they left Laraine to comfort me, which she did admirably.

It wasn't too long before Judy, Laraine's twin sister, arrived with her husband Jim. We filled them in on the latest news and they were so sad for my loss of body parts. Suddenly, out of nowhere, tears just started pouring out of my eyes, and I choked up big time. Laraine was looking the other way, so Judy tapped her on the shoulder and said that she and Jim would step outside for a moment while I recovered my composure. I think Judy was tearing up herself. I did recover, and we later enjoyed some good small talk together. Their added love in the room really did make a difference. Every little bit helps.

After they left, Laraine stayed for the rest of the evening, even as I kept dozing off and coming to again. The nurses kept coming in to check on my pain level which was still, at worst, zero to one on a scale of one to ten. They kept checking because they said they had never had a patient who was not in substantial pain from this type of surgery, especially after the drugs had worn off. I decided I wasn't going to anticipate the obvious and would act as if no pain was imminent. Don't forget, I was a former rugby player.

Later that night, just before I disappeared into a deeper sleep, they checked again and I was still fine. Mentally, I was not in a good place, though. I was bemoaning my situation but realized that I could only go on from where I was, not from where I wanted to be.

VISIONS

The moment I closed my eyes but was not yet asleep, I saw a full blown color image of myself looking down, from far above, on an island. It was a small desert island and was completely filled to the gills with people standing on it from shore to shore, three hundred and sixty degrees. It was standing room only. The image was crystal clear and very detailed, so I was surprised when I realized that all the people were me. I was dressed in every conceivable type of clothing from all ages throughout history. This included styles from many different cultures and multiple types of military uniforms.

    I opened my eyes after a few moments to bring myself back to reality, but on re-closing my eyes I got the same image back immediately. This time I savored the moment and enjoyed the rich spiritual experience I was having. These, surely, must be all of my past lives. The downer of this train of thought was, "Am I in the last hurrahs of this lifetime?" Funnily enough, this didn't bother me in the least. In fact, I was very comfortable with the situation. People who have been resuscitated from a near drowning are said to have experienced bliss during their final gasps of life. I now believe these stories to be true.

That same night, much later, I awoke and lay awake for a short while. On trying to go back to sleep, another vision appeared before my closed eyes, again with the multi-colors, and this time sound. I was going through a real dream while, again, not being quite asleep.

This time I was standing way out of town in the middle of a huge area with about two foot high, swaying grasses. They glistened as they followed the contours of the rolling hills, drawing my eyes to the distant horizon. The sun was bright, and there was a stiff but not uncomfortable breeze. The grasses were hissing as they tossed and rolled in unison with that breeze. Although the scene was quiet, serene and graceful, there was a sense of unease about me. I had no idea why.

Within seconds, I turned to see a monstrous, threatening person barreling toward me at a rapid pace. I was a tad concerned, but not overly, as I watched him (or it) approaching. As he grew closer, I could see he had a large hideous mask over his face, which made him seem more threatening. When he was just a few steps away, I said, "I'm going to protect myself with the HU." When the monster was within arm's reach, I yelled, "Wait a minute. You don't even know the HU," as I ripped off his mask. At this, the individual turned and ran at high speed into the grasses. I understood the monster to be the cancer I was facing, and I understood that if I turned to fight it, I would win.

Soon after this, while still awake but almost asleep, I was a million miles away in space among the stars. About me was a presence that felt as if it spread as far as the eye could see. It sort of had an incredibly thin line but at the same time no line at all. It was as if a being was within my sphere and yet not. I can say that the feeling was of pure divine love.

Was this a message from God? I like to think so, and it was instrumental in my attitude toward this life-threatening disease. Telling people about these visions then wasn't an option, except for Laraine, as I knew they might interpret the stories differently. Also, I didn't want to dissipate any energy that they carried with them. With my spiritual tool bag fully loaded I knew I had a good chance of beating the odds.

The following morning, the first question from my new set of nurses was, "How is your pain level?

The answer was the same: "I have no real pain."

"Let us know right away if that changes," was their retort, as usual. It was almost as if there was a sweepstakes being arranged among the staff as to when I would crack and take some pain medication. I felt I was certainly being looked after by more than physical beings.

I ate a small breakfast before the surgeon reappeared to ask about my well-being. He too was surprised at my lack of pain. Was there a guardian angel in my presence? After he had gone, I recalled the three very real visions from the night before. I was extremely excited about the meanings and the purpose of these visions for me. My confidence and mental wellness took a Saturn rocket-like boost.

Laraine arrived in the early afternoon; I had asked her not to come until then. I wanted to be sure I had settled down from the morning-after rush of sadness I was sure would occur. I needed to look after her well-being as well as my own. Her sadness and fear of losing her somewhat new husband were, I'm sure, in the forefront of her mind.

It was good to see her enter the room; it brought great comfort having her by my side. Just having her hold my hand was a joy unto itself. Again, I dozed a lot, knowing all the while that Laraine was giving all the love I could handle. I was at peace.

At first, as I was recovering, I couldn't walk because I had those tubes wrapped around my legs—y'know the ones that pulsate to keep your blood flowing as you lie, more or less still, in the bed. They felt weird.

Flowers kept arriving from all kinds of people, joining the beautiful ones Laraine had placed close to me. They were accompanied by well-wishing cards of love. Later, Judy and Jim came by again, as did three sets of friends. Although it was tiring to have visitors, they really helped my psyche. They were politely quiet as they spoke in whispered voices and didn't outstay their welcome. It felt good to be loved.

For all of you who wonder what to do for friends who are suffering, my advice is to let them know, if nothing else, that they are loved. It makes a huge difference in these circumstances. You don't even have to say anything. Be there, and they will know.

ON THE THIRD DAY

On day three, a different kind of help entered my world—a person of great service and very significant. She was to show me how to empty my latest friend, the colostomy bag. I was half with the program and didn't really get the gist of all that she demonstrated, but I figured all would be repeated before I left the hospital. This woman was incredibly loving and kind, especially with such a messy job to perform and teach.

It was at this time that I learned how horrifically smelly old dried blood can be. As my neck snapped into violent convulsions and tried to depart from the rest of my body, the nurse sprayed a mist over the area. The relief to the nostrils was a joy only surpassed by going to Disney World for the first time. I was to learn that this dried blood would take quite a while to finally clear my intestines completely. I assumed the painters would be by later to redo the peeling paint on the walls and ceiling from the smell. They should put that stuff into sprayers to ward off street attackers. It surely outshines bear and pepper spray by a wide margin.

Also on day three, I turned over and felt something fall out of my back. Laraine was there and saw it come out; I didn't know I'd had anything in there as I had been on my back the whole time. It turns out I had an epidural attached. It's like a permanent drip feed into the back to administer drugs. Did it explain my freedom from pain? I wondered why I hadn't felt it there, but I suppose the drugs themselves took that feeling away.

The nurse said that now, for sure, I would feel pain, but it never did happen. I wonder if that nurses' sweepstakes is still going.

Sadly it was time for Laraine to leave, and I watched her until she disappeared round the doorway. It was at this point I was allowed to get up and carefully take a shower. I was scared to fully see, for the first time, my attachment in all its glory. I was so nervous at the thought of just seeing it.

It wasn't a pretty picture. My surgery site was still very red, purple, blue and yellow, and the large metal staples made me look like Frankenstein. It took me forever just to get up the nerve to wash around that area and, on completing the shower, to dry that same area. It was all a little too much for my mind to comprehend, but I made it back to the safety of my bed without incident. Sleep was once again clawing at my body.

I lay there pondering my future for quite a while as reality hit. We had a phrase in the navy for when things were going downhill, for whatever reason, on a personal level: *Death, death where is thy sting?* It was appropriate for how I was thinking in this wretched hour of my life.

The following morning, though, led me to a very different perspective. After being poked, prodded, and questioned, I was in a trance-like state mentally and started to look into myself, I mean really look into myself, and the situation. I knew I needed to make a quantum shift in my approach to the rest of my life. How was I going to handle my mind and turn this new experience, *challenge* if you like, into something positive?

One idea immediately jumped to the fore: what if I owned this cancer? If I owned it, it couldn't possibly own me.

I liked this. I decided I was going to own the cancer, train it and control it, and then kick it out. Of course, I would still need the medications and cancer center to guide and support me, but I would also gather myself a team of positive ideas and fight the good fight. I was going to win and then encourage other people to fight and win–or at least go down fighting.

This uplifted me enormously, and I was feeling better about myself. I still had some low moments, but I had a future to look forward to and was going to make the most of it. My heart and stomach started to feel less fluttery, and the weight on my shoulders felt much lighter. I had a long way to go but the light at the end of the tunnel was not another train coming, for sure.

Day three was the day I was allowed to walk for the first time, albeit excruciatingly slowly, more of a shuffle really, around the hallways outside of my room. I dodged in and out of various rooms to try and uplift my neighboring patients with a smile, short chat, and a joke or two—that is, until a staff member saw me coming out of a room and had a conniption fit. Apparently this isn't done for various reasons such as that I might catch whatever they had, privacy (duh) and, oh I don't know. The list went on so long that I logged out of planet earth for a while. Anyway, I didn't do that again.

Days four and five were a doddle. I knew the routine and I knew all the staff. I still felt weak and slept a lot but was feeling more settled. Around 9 o'clock in the evening on day five, the surgeon came into my room. He gave me a once over check and asked if I would like to go home. Actually, I really didn't want to at this late hour, but I said yes.

    It seemed to all happen in about five minutes but was, I'm sure, a lot longer. My catheter was removed. Laraine had been called to come and pick me up, my stuff was packed, and I was on my way. Look out world, here I come.

The whirlwind came to an abrupt halt when I tried to get out of the car. Even with Laraine's help, it took forever to extract me from the seat and then go up three steps to the main floor of the house, then up another eight steps in our tri-level house and into bed. This was going to be a process.

KARMA BUSTER

Before going to sleep one afternoon I asked my spiritual guide if there was a particular karmic reason why I had contracted cancer. If there was, could I be shown it in a dream or during a soul travel experience? During my deep sleep that same afternoon I got a crystal clear answer.

I had one of those lifelike dreams with sound and multi-colors, and it seemed like it was actually happening in the real physical world we live in. I dreamed I was a soldier way back in medieval times. You know, I'm sure, about those battles where there were thousands of soldiers on each side that just walked or charged into each other. Both armies were coming down a hillside to meet at the bottom of a valley. I was in the second row with a very long lance that went over the shoulders of the front rank and into the front rank of the opposition when we closed in on each other.

The dream fast forwarded to individual fighting, and I was coming down a narrow path on the hill. Lying down on the path and severely injured was a soldier of the opposing army. I still had my lance and poised to thrust it into his body. He was already out of the action and no use to man or beast as far as fighting was concerned. His bulging eyes stared at me as he begged for mercy and to live another day. I totally ignored his pleas for help and skewered him to death, no mercy shown.

This is where it got really interesting. The place where my spear entered his body was exactly where my stoma protruded. The dream ended at this juncture, and I woke up feeling great remorse for that enemy soldier. It was so real I could have touched it. This couldn't be a coincidence. I had asked for a reason for the cancer and the dream came that same afternoon.

Funnily enough, this helped tremendously in my recovery. I knew why I had cancer and the colostomy and felt reassured that I was merely paying off karma and that I would be okay in the end. (*In the end*—I couldn't help it.) I was almost happy that I had cancer and was grateful to God for being given the opportunity to burn off such a large error in judgment in a previous life. Isn't life grand, if you don't weaken? I do want to be clear though; don't wish for cancer to burn off karma. My happiness had a narrow window in which to operate in that vein.

RECOVERY TIME

I am not sure what the word *bedridden* means. When I was in bed all the time, I had not got *rid* of the bed but was, alas, bedridden nonetheless. My main problem was being able to sleep and rest only on my back. Any pressure from lying on my side was painful and, to be honest, scary. Naturally, turning onto my stomach was out of the question.

Because of the huge amount of dried blood that had coagulated in my intestines from the surgery, any excretion was hard, solid and large. This made for terrible pain, which made me cry out involuntarily.

During the night, when Laraine was by my side, I worried that she would be worried. I spent a lot of time trying to protect her from such concerned thinking. Even all these years later, I'm still not sure if that was the right way to go.

The wound care center at the hospital showed me how to change the colostomy bag, which didn't have to be changed too often at first. I wasn't eating that much, and the intestine was starting out empty. I was afraid to change my new friend on my own and went to the hospital for the first four times of changing my bag.

On the fourth visit they told me the insurance would only allow five demonstrations. This was a good thing as I needed to bite the bullet and change it myself, and alone. I had never shied away from a challenge before. Why was I doing it now?

The process, at first, was more difficult than it would be later as I needed to cut a circle out of the sticky patch that went onto my skin around the stoma. Once the stoma had settled down and reached a point where it wouldn't change size or shape, I would be able to buy ready-cut flanges. The colostomy bag clipped onto the flange, which was the easy part.

The first time I attempted this on my own at home, I readied myself at the sink in the bathroom. Laraine called out to me on three occasions during the two and a half hour process. She was very worried for me and wondered what the heck was going on. At the hospital it took but fifteen minutes. I was a little depressed about how much time it took and was thinking, *Is this the situation for the rest of my life?*

While one has the stoma exposed with the bag off, there is always the danger of a discharge as no muscles are there to control any output. Oh boy! This was going to be miserable. *Come on, Barry, I told myself. This is not the attitude that is going to get you through this. Not a lot of new opportunities are easy from the get-go. Pull yourself together. There are no problems, only solutions to find.* That mantra—There are no problems, only solutions to find—had been with me the whole of my working life, taught to me by my very first chief on my first ship in the Royal Navy.

The nurses at the Wound Center also showed me how to clean the expensive and reusable bags in the toilet. After a month of doing that, I quit and used a fresh bag each time. The cleaning was time-consuming, messy and tricky. I was affluent enough to cover the cost of extra bags not covered by insurance each month. This eased my concerns and worries, and as time marched on I got quicker and quicker at the changing of the guard.

Eventually I could buy the pre-cut flanges and things got better and better. *See how that works?* I thought. *Be patient, keep working at it, and do the best you can.* I often thought of the millions of people who were so much worse off than I and still living long and cheerful lives. It felt as if they were showing me the way. Now I could spend more time on beating the ogre still in my body, the cancer.

I have an ongoing exchange with some of my friends that I reiterate from time to time. I believe that if a thing's worth doing, it's worth doing badly. My argument is that if the best you can do with any new experience is poorly, it is still the best you can do. If you keep doing it anyway, you will gradually improve. Soon you might even become the best at doing it, whatever it may be. Do you know how many rockets exploded or went awry before we put a man on the moon? Well, neither do I, actually, but I know there were a lot.

The ankle biter across the road was barking and barking every day. It was tied up at the front of the driveway, the poor mite. Laraine bravely went over there and explained how annoying the barking was to not only the neighborhood but to a very sick husband trying to rest and recuperate. It was impossible for me to sleep for any length of time, slowing my return to normality. The neighbors must have taken the hint as Ruffles, the noise machine, was quiet from then on.

I started spending time in the recliner downstairs. Getting down there and lowering my carcass into the chair was tricky and slow but worth the effort. Normality was my next goal in life.

Eventually I asked Laraine if we could walk around the block, and she agreed. It is a very large block, maybe three quarters of a mile. I needed to hold onto Laraine, and my steps were not even a foot long. Actually, they were more like shuffle-and-slides than steps, and the journey required three rest stops. Approaching about halfway, I was feeling I couldn't make it home. I kept this to myself and soldiered on until the marathon ended back in my recliner. This brought home to me the enormous effort my recovery would take, but didn't bring my optimism down.

The next day we did the same journey and it was much better.

Week four saw me getting a port put into my chest above the heart, which required an operation. The port was a disc placed under the skin four inches below the collar bone with a tube running into my artery just before it entered my heart. A special needle that looked like a fish hook was to be poked into this disc each time I went to the cancer center for my juice, i.e. poison. Yes, chemo was on the horizon. The port saved my arms from being torn up by IVs going into them week after week. After it was in place, my whole chest was black, red, blue, and purple from the blood under my skin. I looked like a coloring book that had been dropped in water. The swelling around the surgical site was also horrendous, but this was one of the best moves made for my overall well-being for the near future.

I had been getting a pay check from my job as I had three weeks of vacation available. On the fourth week, I got a phone call from John, my boss, who told me my pay check was waiting for me in the office. I told him that I had already received my third and final check the previous week. He said, rather more firmly, "Your pay check is in the office." I repeated my response, and so did he. This wonderful person and his wife, who was an important and integral part of the company, had decided they were going to pay me for the whole five weeks off. They were both very good to me, and I will be eternally grateful to them for that.

On week five I was walking around normally, for the most part, and could operate at almost maximum speed. I revisited the cancer center for further instructions as to my future treatment at this juncture. Chemotherapy was the first step, which I started on the sixth week.

I was to have a belt around my waist with chemo in it, along with a pump. The pump would shoot chemo into me via a tube and into that port, which took the fish hook shaped needle. This insertion of juice would be administered every fifteen minutes, 24/7, for the next five weeks.

BACK TO WORK

Going back to work was going to be intimidating. I now had that colostomy bag to negotiate while using a Port-O-Let, as well as the chemo belt to contend with. And I knew I would have radiation when I finished with the chemo belt. That would be another hurdle to jump.

I am going to jump straight to that first day of radiation. It was like entering another world within my new world. The staff members in the radiation department were unbelievable in every way. I had to expose my delicate areas each day as the death ray machine did its work. It didn't take long, maybe twenty minutes, but they made the experience as pleasant as possible. We swapped jokes and funny stories and also had some more serious moments. Brian, the leader of the two associates, told me one day that as far as he could see, negative-thinking patients probably died from cancer eighty-five percent of the time whereas positive people succeeded eighty-five percent of the time. That being said, though, some positive people discovered their cancer when it was too rampant in their bodies and could not be rescued, despite their positive thinking. I was a very positive thinker, so this boosted my confidence and gave me even more hope.

My time for the rads was first thing in the morning at 7.30 am so I could get in a full day's work. I was radiated, juiced up and ready to go.

My first day back involved a lot of tears as my co-workers welcomed me with open arms, especially the two bosses, John and his wife. The next surprise was just around the corner, literally. The boss came to the truck with me, which was unusual, but I didn't really think about it. Before I got in, he said, "Let me show you something," and walked to the back of the truck. On lifting the top half of the hinged opening and dropping the tailgate, he pulled out the floor of the truck.

He had installed a pull out bed so that I didn't have to climb into the truck to retrieve whatever it was I needed. He knew it would be tricky for me with the colostomy. How much more could this man do for me? He and his wife were the most wonderful people I could have had as bosses. I am pretty sure it cost at least $800.00 to have this done. I was gobsmacked and just about shook his hand off.

It was time to head for a job site and start a new beginning of my working life. At the house we were to wire, I let the lads roll out the equipment while I studied the drawings. I always spent a while walking a house carrying the drawings with me to assess the skills of the architect. Architects are not electricians, and I would always adjust the layout, especially on the larger houses that had not been rubber stamped. With the custom houses, the superintendent would generally get the home owner to walk with me. This way I could explain to them why I thought the lighting or three and four way switches and receptacles should be changed or added.

Day one went without a hitch although I was really tired and was glad to see the hands of time bringing the day to a close. The main reason the day was okay was because I spent most of it marking the two-by-fours for the apprentices to know where to nail on the different specific boxes I needed. The next day I would be tested to a far greater degree.

When I got home Laraine was waiting with bated breath wondering how I had fared on my first day. It was then that I realized how much more difficult it was for her than for me in some ways. I think she had spent the whole day worrying about how I was getting along.

Laraine had spent a good portion of the day cooking a very special meal for me. It was one of my favorites, salmon, along with yellow, red and bright green vegetables. She made it look so inviting because she knew how hard it was for me to eat. The chemo will do that to you, destroy your appetite.

When I put the salmon in my mouth and started to chew it was like eating tin foil. I couldn't eat it.

I remember resting my head in my hands with my elbows on the table and sobbing my heart out. Laraine didn't immediately know what was up and rushed to my side, holding my shoulders. I couldn't speak to tell her what was going on for quite a while. When I eventually calmed down and told her, she totally understood, telling me, "It's okay." Well, to me, it wasn't okay, and I felt awful. Everything Laraine did for me was with love, and she soaked up so much emotion which she hid from me. I was bushed and made it to the recliner before slumping into sleep for a couple of hours. I awoke to Laraine holding my hand which, again, was so soothing.

At work the chemo belt prevented me from wearing my tool belt, so I would carry it in my hand from place to place. This belt of poison that, nevertheless, was saving my life also stopped me from sleeping very easily. When I went to the cancer center for a top up and battery change, I explained this to them. The doc gave me some Ambien to help me sleep.

BREAKDOWN

That first night I swallowed the magic pill and slept rather well. The day went okay and on returning home I walked up the driveway, where Laraine was waiting to greet me. She said, "How was your day today?" with a great big smile. I looked at her and broke down into a major crying event. I couldn't stop sobbing to the point where I could barely breathe. She got me into the house and eventually calmed me down. I didn't know what was happening.

Wisely, Laraine thought it might be the Ambien. I didn't see why that would be as I had been perfectly okay all day. It was strange that I would break down as soon as I got home.

The next day I was really down all day and had trouble maintaining any semblance of cheerfulness. This was so unusual for me, even with the cancer. After I got home we went to the cancer center and told them what was going on. They immediately told me to stop taking the Ambien and try some different pills instead. I forget what they were, but they did the trick as far as the sleep went.

The next day I felt all right, as I did the following evening. I was back to normal. Apparently Ambien can trigger a particular reaction in some people—I think they said one in forty—and they go into a deep depression. I had never suffered from depression before, but this experience gave me a lesson on how to empathize with people who do. I realized you are completely out of control of your emotions.

I was starting to wonder how many more lessons this cancer situation was going to teach me before I was cured. Yes, cured. That is where I was headed, and I vowed to stay positive and stay upbeat.

A VOICE OUT OF THE BLUE

It was time for my first multi-hour chemo indoctrination; the 24/7 bag was complete. I nervously walked into the room which I had previously been shown. It had five very large, very comfortable recliners with a regular chair beside each.

I was surprised to see a familiar face. A good friend, Mary, from my spiritual path, Eckankar, was sitting next to her husband, who had a large needle in his arm instead of a port in his chest like me. We'd had no idea they were going through this trauma. Although we had a quick exchange of conversation, the nurses needed me to sit and be prepped for infusion. We did speak at length later in the week, though.

After "hello" pleasantries from the other patients, I felt a little quiet and nestled into an empty recliner. Two young nurses approached and immediately put me at ease, as much as was humanly possible at this point in time. They explained how they were going to insert this strangely shaped fishhook-like needle into my port. They continued by telling me how long it would likely take to infuse the multiple—yes, multiple—bags of chemo and how the chemo might affect me during the following week. Everybody has a different experience, they said. They were so kind and gentle, even in their body language and wording. They didn't treat me like I was just another patient on the conveyor belt—you know, like, "Let's hook him up and go read at the desk." Everything was done and said as if I was the most special person and only person in their work life.

They prepped my port with a cleansing antiseptic wipe and told me the next part might hurt a little. I was to take a deep breath and blow out as they inserted the needle. It was like baiting the hook before swishing the fishing line into the water. The problem was, I was the bait. I didn't feel the needle too much and settled down for a three hour fuel transfer.

The other patients were a fairly quiet group, using only intermittent polite conversation, and I let them have their peace. Two were dozing and others whispered to their spouses. Laraine and I followed suit and the scene was set. Eventually my fishing, fuel transfer line was disengaged in a like manner to the hook up, and I was free to move about the cabin.

As I was leaving, the wonderful receptionist at the reception desk was chatting with the social worker assigned to the cancer center. My appearance gave June, the social worker, the opportunity to address me about a support group. The group met every Tuesday from 5:30 to 7:30 p.m. I told her that I most likely wouldn't be joining as I am not a group type of guy. Besides, I was comfortable with my cancer and had a great support group of my own. This group included my wife Laraine, local family, Eckankar as my spiritual path, my electrical company, and a host of friends that were by my side. I politely left it at that and headed for the exit.

I had radiation in the morning, and so when I got home that evening I ate a little of something Laraine had prepared and nestled into my recliner for the rest of the evening.

The next day I felt pretty good and really didn't feel any effects from the chemo. My work day went as normal, though very tiring, and I got home with no real problems. Day two of post chemo was a tad more tiring, and on day three, Thursday, things went a little awry. Around mid–afternoon, after dragging for an hour or more, I was ascending the stairs from the basement. About half-way up the stairs I suddenly couldn't take another step. When I called out to my apprentice, he came and virtually carried me to the top. My boss and Laraine were called, and Laraine came and picked me up and took me home. I was overcome with sadness as we trundled into the house. I was devastated.

The evening was quiet for me as I mulled over the situation. Was I going to be able to continue to work? I wasn't sure how Laraine felt, but I suspected that she was feeling sad and was worried about my state of mind.

This is where things get tricky for the care giver. They don't want to give away their feelings, and the patient doesn't want to give away theirs. Honesty is not prevalent at this stage of the game because we are trying too hard to protect each other. Folks, don't do this! Let it all hang out and totally share your feelings and thoughts from the beginning. We later realized that being open with each other helped rather than hindered our situation. This was another lesson in life that both of us learned.

Laraine begged me not to go to work on Friday. I told her I had to, for my survival. I was going to smash my way through this thicket and come out the other end unscathed. As she kissed me goodbye and waved, I wondered, "What is her state of mind? How is she feeling? How worried is she?" Thinking back, going to work may have been a selfish thing to do, but at the time it was what I needed to do. I made it through the day and was wrapped in Laraine's arms as I stepped into the kitchen that afternoon.

The two day weekend was spent chilling out and recuperating for the next week. On Monday my refueling station was waiting for me again as they re-gassed me for the next round. I had told Laraine she need not come with me to the cancer center as I would go straight from work. I don't think she liked that very much, but it all made sense. I would leave work early, mid-afternoon, every Monday from then on to soak up the juice.

At every treatment at the cancer center, Pauline, the oncologist, would step into the room with the patients and chat with us, both individually and as a group. She always had tons of snacks and goodies in the small kitchen area for anybody to nibble on. This she paid for out of her own pocket. After a couple of weeks I would bring in special treats also as I was still earning a good wage and wanted to chip in for the group.

The same people were always there, except when somebody had completed their doses. Of course, there were also the few who had decided to pass on to their next soul experience.

I couldn't continue with the relatively silent structure for too long and ramped up the chatter as time went on. Eventually we were sharing stories of all kinds. There were humorous, sad, scandalous, and really interesting anecdotes and, as we opened up more generously, some more juicy and saucy ones. We laughed a lot and had a good old time; even the nurses joined in the fun and told some good stories of their own. They never divulged any stories of past or present patients, of course, which was probably a shame; I'll bet they had a tale or two to tell.

I was checking out at registration one day when something phenomenal happened. The subject of the cancer support group came up with a couple of other people in the vicinity. As I was eavesdropping, I said to myself, *Ha, not for me.* The next thing I knew, a voice—not in my head but physically there—said, "You may not need them but they may need you." There was a piercing sound in my ears as goose bumps shimmied across my skin and cooled my body. I looked around and nobody else was there, other than the two others discussing the group. I drove home in a bit of a haze and thought about it all that evening. Now what?

THE SUPPORT GROUP

Could it have been a spirit or God speaking to me? My spiritual path is known as the Path of Spiritual Freedom, so it was my choice whether or not I followed the voice's suggestion. Should I go ahead and give the group a shot? What was the harm? I could always bail out if I didn't care for it.

The next day, I walked through the sliding glass doors at 5:15 p.m. and came across June setting up the chairs. There were three other cancer patients already waiting, but they were a little too weak to assist her, so I helped. The hospital had delivered juices, coffee, and tea along with sandwiches for the group, which was the normal practice every week. I thought that was very classy of the hospital, as it was not something they had to do.

The room included two couches and multiple chairs that were fairly large and well-cushioned. On the far wall was a very nice stone fireplace with a large mantelpiece. The setting had a warm, cozy feel to it.

I chose a chair and waited for the proceedings to begin. Slowly people arrived and immediately came over and introduced themselves. Everybody else knew each other so it was clear when a fresh face was upon them. June started the meeting and gave a very nice opening statement. Then one of the group members started to reveal how he was doing and how he had felt this last week. He gave some very personal descriptions involving private parts about what the treatment was doing to him. Then he calmly looked to his left for the next person to speak.

This continued on around the room with participants equally sharing, in gay abandon, all and sundry about their cancer, where it was and what it was doing. The unabashed explanations of these people's private parts and conditions were quite overwhelming. They were very comfortable with each other and shared all to the fullest. It was customary to have the newbies go last, presumably to give them the chance to see how the land lay and to accustom themselves to total honesty and unabridged regurgitation of prognoses. Okay, my turn.

My first words were, "Oh dear, I think I have come to the wrong group. I thought this was an AA meeting. Hi, my name is Barry and I'm an alcoholic." Well, everybody burst out laughing as they already knew I was a cancer patient. I realized I was among a great group of people and this was right for me.

Three months into chemo and having finished my radiation long ago, a man called David, the same age as me, came into the group. His level of stage four colon cancer was the same as mine, as was his treatment and course of action. He had received his new friend, the colostomy, and radiation and chemo were on the agenda. This isn't a criticism of David by any means, but, his mental approach to the enemy, cancer, was very different than that of most of the group. Now we were not all clicking our heels and jumping for joy, but we were mostly very positive thinking. One person, Colin, had stage four pancreatic cancer and, along with his wife, was still extremely upbeat.

David, it turns out, was let go by his parking lot night cleaning company. Without this job, he had lost his medical insurance. He could not afford private insurance so was dead in the water as far as proper care was concerned. He could not get a port in his chest like me and therefore had to suffer getting a large needle inserted into his wrist every week. This may not seem a big deal to the uninitiated, but after several weeks his arms looked like a four-times-a-day junkie's. It became difficult for the nurses to find a decent vein.

His and my chemo cost about ten thousand dollars a week, and that is not a typo. Naturally, it was impossible for him to keep up with any payment. His radiation had already put him in the poor house—actually, it had cost him his house. David's longtime live-in companion had left him, and he could not find another job. David and I had exactly the same disease with the exact same severity and treatment, but our lives were so very different. Our conditions were definitely not the same when you looked below the surface. The difference between the insured and the uninsured is enormous in every way.

He could hardly be faulted for his attitude toward the cancer and life in general, considering his situation. He did take some subtle, underhanded, poorly disguised flak from some group members about his attitude. I quietly jumped to his defense, along with three others who, with me, had become leaders of the group at this point. We didn't want him to stop coming to the support group, especially as we were all he had to lean on. I reminded the participants that we were a support group, not a guidance or judgmental group. Whatever people wanted to do, we supported them in it, suicide maybe being the exception. That we would hand over to the experts.

Sometimes we had a guest speaker, musician, or even, sometimes, an oncology doctor or specialist to speak to us. Generally, though, the Four Musketeers informally steered the group, along with June, our guiding force and leader of general well-being. I always believed that June knew everything that went on between, around, over and through every action and thought within the walls of the cancer center. She was incredibly perceptive and a fully aware person who kept her finger on the pulse of things at all times.

I remember one very long suffering person finally trying marijuana to alleviate the pain that she endured. Some of the members sort of snubbed her; at least that is how she felt. I have to interject that they were the more religious ones. I chatted with her for a while after the meeting and gave her my full support. I'm pretty sure she and June had some consultations about it, too. Anyway, some of us made sure that the marijuana lady kept her head high and was comfortable with the group. Some people, though, still looked down upon her for smoking the forbidden weed. (Nowadays, in Colorado, it is legal for recreational purposes. For medical reasons it has been legal for much longer.)

It was, after a while, getting tougher and tougher to maintain my strength and perform at work, but perform I did. I certainly earned my pay, but it was hard. Laraine sometimes pleaded with me to give it up because she saw how I looked when I got home. Slumping in the recliner was becoming the norm. The wonderful, appetizing, and colorful meals she cooked made it easier on me, and with her support I knew I could keep going. Work was one of the main lifelines to my success, and I needed it.

One of my main apprentices, Casey Shupe, certainly helped a tremendous amount. If he saw me lifting heavy equipment or starting to go into an attic, he would jump all over me and take over that task.

When I said, "No," he took charge and adamantly told me off. His camaraderie, compassion, and grace were exemplary, beyond the norm for sure.

One main job site I was working on was run by a family. Vicky and Gary Mackey were the developers and in charge of everything with Vicky being the superintendent and financial guru. Gary ran the heavy machinery along with the son, Bryon. The daughter, Robin, as with the mother, carried out multiple other tasks as well. I write about this because the whole family was always keeping one eye open for me. They were absolutely wonderful and very caring about my welfare. Was I looked after or what? I don't know what I would have done without them.

We really had some fun times during the re-fueling process, in other words, chemo. I was normally the last one to have the needle and fueling hoses hooked up. Therefore, I was the last to leave around six o'clock. One winter afternoon, when I arrived in the infusion room, I was wearing five layers of clothing. As I started to peel off the top coat, somebody started singing the "stripper" melody and clapping. Well, everybody started up with the tune then, and I began gyrating and slowly removed the next item. This I swung around my head and threw it across the floor. I finally got down to my tee shirt and peeled that off also. That one had to go back on, though, as it was too cool in the room for a bare chest. Anyway, I didn't want to get everybody too excited.

Three huge teddy bears named Faith, Hope and Charity sat on top of some cabinets looking down on everybody, and I swear I saw them clapping and chanting with everybody else. Laraine and I had bought the three bears just before Christmas, on sale at one of the big box stores. When I told the store register lady why I was buying them and who for, she called the manager over ,and she knocked even more money off our ticket. Is this a great country or what?

Everybody was laughing and having a good time. The oncologist dashed in to see what the heck was going on, along with any staff member who was close enough to make it in time.

However, all good things must come to an end, and in went the needle as out rushed my breath. I was starting to have trouble getting the chemo to pump into my body and needed to move my arms around in all kinds of crazy positions. It was taking much longer to drain the bags than when I started. It wasn't a big deal, though, and we coped with the situation.

In typical fashion for me, I would often try to crawl backwards in the recliner away from the nurse as she approached with the needle and goop. I would say, "No, no, please, no more, please," or words to that effect. They always laughed and stuck me anyway.

TURNOVERS WITH SADNESS AND JOY

The faces started to change more often during my chemo sessions. Some people were not on such a long regimen as me. Some had been there long before I came by. As each new person came along, we welcomed them into the fold. There was a quieter and more private area if somebody needed to be by themselves for a while.

Although I am making light of our situation in the chemo room that day, there were many less fun times, and often there were times of sadness. At these times, we would have a more gracious and quiet, loving moment to listen and empathize with whoever it was who needed it, especially with somebody new.

Well into my time with the support group, I was telling everyone how, a few days earlier, I had really been tearful. When driving home one night, my colostomy burst open, and there was a heck of a mess for me to manage while still needing to drive to the house. I was really bummed out and remonstrating about the condition I was going to be in for the rest of my life. I was cursing my luck and went downhill fast.

I went on to tell the group how I recovered and got back to normal mentally, ending my talk with, "Shit happens." Everybody burst out laughing and cheering. It had been just an off-the-cuff remark, so I had no way of expecting that reaction.

There was a new elderly lady who had come to the group that night. I spoke to her after the session, giving a personal welcome, and listening to a deeper version of her woes. I liked to do that to the newcomers when it was appropriate and possible. A few weeks later, she told the group that, like myself, she wasn't a group type person and wasn't sure she really wanted to join us. But when she heard me say, "Shit happens," she knew she was with the right people. She became a solid, permanent member.

I had just blurted that comment out, but it had made a difference. You never know when or how you are going to be used by God to help somebody. That has to be spirit pulling the strings doesn't it?

This lady, Ruth, had been diagnosed with stage four cervical cancer. She had been fighting cancer for a long time, and the doctors had told her they couldn't do any more for her and to go home and get her affairs in order. They reckoned that Ruth had, at most, six months to live.

Well, Ruth was tough. I remember one night when she came to the group all excited and puffed up. A couple of days earlier, she had gone outside of her isolated house in the country and got a big surprise. As she turned the corner a huge black bear was a few feet from her. Ruth shouted and screamed at the also startled bear and ran for the back door. Obviously, she made it because there she was relaying the event.

This very strong-willed and powerfully-minded person wasn't letting the doctors' prognosis be the final word. This fighting 'Tasmanian Devil' buckled down and started researching alternative medicine. After a while, she started taking a seed of some exotic plant in the Amazon forest. It could have been the spit of the endangered lesser spotted yellow tongued toad, for all I know. I'm not sure. But after several months, she was completely clear of cancer and lived a strong and much longer life than anticipated.

One of the doctors at the clinic was asked to be the guest speaker one evening. He wasn't my particular oncologist, thank goodness. If he had been, I would probably have sought a different one. He gave us some good information on the newest ways of battling cancer, but he gave me the impression that we were meant to be getting our lives in order. I presume you know what I mean by that. Yeah, as in "You don't have much time left."

My main question for him was, "Do you believe being positive and tapping into your spiritual beliefs can help to cure ones cancer?"

He categorically said, "No."

This totally railed against all of my senses. I gave him both barrels and then reloaded. How dare he impose his beliefs on us? It was as if he had donned large hob-nailed boots and trodden all over our delicately built, artistically fabricated tapestry of hope. He really did think that it was purely one hundred percent the drugs and only the drugs that decided whether we lived or died.

Talk about a single vision, narrow minded nonbeliever. After my double barreled rebuff and chafing, he did not relent or step back one iota. Some people are clever, some intellectual and some have common sense and mojo. I'm sure this doctor was very clever, but I will leave it there.

I believe we need to use every means available to our psyche and physical body to attack this disease. It certainly worked for me, so why not others? Luckily, all the nurses and certainly my oncologist were always encouraging us to use all avenues and weapons open to us. We didn't need his negative waves. His comments were vanquished by the group, and our tapestry of hope survived.

SAYING GOODBYES

As time rolled on, I was getting used to being tired in the evenings. It became a way of life, and Laraine and I both accepted it. It was like we took a sabbatical from our regular life. Judy and Jim, the "outlaws," were still extremely supportive and super kind. I love them dearly for their consistent words of encouragement.

We had a saying in the navy: If you are cool, calm, and collected while everybody about you is in a panic, you are not fully aware of the situation. Keeping that in mind, it was time for me to be brought down to earth a little. Although the group was superbly uplifting, there were times when reality hurt. Sometimes beloved members lost the fight for remaining on this physical plane and retired to the next. I could look at it as a blessing for them to be relieved of this painful world, and I did. However, that didn't make their leaving any easier, maybe because I was selfish and wanted their company even if they were in so much pain. My feelings were mixed; I was happy for them and sad for myself.

I often wonder why nobody wants to die or is so afraid to die. The churches preach how wonderful God and heaven are, but nobody wants to go there. It's like not wanting to go to Disney World for the first time because it is so enjoyable.

The experiences of losing our precious friends did percolate through the support group from time to time. This really brought home the fact that I was in more trouble than I likely realized. That stalwart old saying, *One day at a time,* came into full force then. On these occasions of great loss, June would light a candle, and we had a moment of silence for the deceased. We then had a section of the meeting when anybody who wanted to could share their feelings.

One of the Fab Four, Don, my very best support friend, passed into the next world one day. I was totally shocked and hurt more than was normal. It came about so rapidly, as if he suddenly hit an off ramp and slid down an embankment. After the candle had been lit and the moment of silence had passed, everybody looked at me. I was too distraught to speak at that moment and waved my hand from side to side. June immediately asked if anyone else wanted to share. As time went by and more people spoke, I regained my composure and managed to swallow the knot in my throat. Don was such a standard setter for all who came. The bar he set was never too high and never too low and was adjustable to whoever was sharing in any moment of time. Anyway, I did manage to share my personal feelings and give Don my own heartfelt eulogy.

TEA AND CRUMPETS, ANYONE?

During one of the summer months June asked the support group if we would like an outside meeting on the patio next to the foyer. We all agreed and the following week when we arrived, everything was set up for our fresh air excursion from the norm. June had also arranged with the hospital to put on a barbecue type spread for us. Everybody was amazed at the layout and we settled in for the duration of the meet.

Five minutes into the first person speaking, a helicopter flew by and was circling overhead as if looking for somebody or something. We later found out a moose was in the area and needed to be tranquilized and returned to the mountains. We, of course, couldn't hear ourselves speak. Eventually chopper man decided to leave the area. That was great, but not long after that the grounds crew spent the next half hour mowing the lawns surrounding the center. We were now all wondering if meeting outside was such a good idea. That thought was confirmed as a "No, it's not a good idea" when the lawn mowers left and the hedge trimmers and lawn edgers started work. By now we were all laughing at the situation, and everybody who could helped get all the food and furniture back inside the foyer area. That great idea turned into a catastrophe and was chalked up as a hilarious evening to remember. We did have a good time and appreciated the hospital going the extra mile for us yet again.

When I got to the group meeting one afternoon, June called me into the office. There was to be a fund raiser dinner at the hospital in a couple of weeks, and she wondered if I would be willing to make a speech. Naturally, I jumped at the chance as that is what I love to do.

The dinner was well-attended by a large number of the hoity-toity of the community—you know, the money bags in town who needed a tax break. Part of my job was to help them decide that the cancer center was their best dumping ground. I really don't mean to disparage these people because they are a vital part of any society. Their generosity is to be greatly and graciously accepted to the max.

On the day of the races I wore my best suit along with my bow tie. Several hospital dignitaries stepped up for their speeches before I was called to the fore. I explained to them the feel of the cancer center and how all of the staff members from janitor to surgeon were exemplary in their care and understanding of us patients. I wanted them to understand the importance of not only the medical side of the center but the caring side as well. I thought that explaining other aspects of what the center is about might lengthen their arms so they could go deeper into those pockets. My mind was working on how I could hold them upside down and shake them by the ankles to drain out those last few loose coins.

The evening went very well, and I got a chance to speak to the mayor and some councilors along with other members of high society. I also managed to get in a few words with the hospital director and CEO. I so wanted them to know how much we appreciated how the whole cancer crew treated us—like royalty.

I never did find out how much money was donated or promised, but I am guessing it was a lot. Anyway, I had a good time and enjoyed partying with the toffs and bourgeoisie.

The other "munchies" time of year came around at Christmas. Each patient, plus one, was invited, along with all the staff plus one, to a Christmas dinner. This was held at the hospital and was always quite a lavish meal. The participants included anybody who was not only an active cancer patient but also anyone who still attended the support group.

The meal they served was always amazing with salad, a main course that consisted of various choices of meats with all the trimmings, along with multiple deserts—certainly not a let's-do-just-enough-to-keep-them-happy kind of evening. There was even music supplied by a local band or musician. I'm telling you right now, cancer can be a blast. I still wouldn't recommend it just to have great camaraderie and free meals every now and again, but it's a close call.

By now I was in total control of how the chemo sessions were going to go. I speak in jest, of course. Although some of the guests had a tough time, it was good to see the spirit in even the weakest person, physically that is.

I learned a lot about when and when not to jest with an individual. I found I could start out with love and consideration and then slowly turn the conversation into a more jovial event. On a rare occasion, this wasn't possible, and I would go with the flow and end with wishing them well and hoping they had a better week than the one they just experienced. I found that lightly holding their hand or just touching their hand as I disengaged from the chat seemed to comfort them. I think it was because it showed I cared, I mean really cared, because I did.

One weekly consistent message I wouldn't let go of was the sign on the wall as we left the area to go to the registration desk. It said, "Check Out Here." Every week I would tell them that the sign was totally inappropriate as we patients were not about to give up our lives and check out. After a while, just as I was about to say it again, they would say, "I know, I know, you are not about to check out yet." We would laugh and go on our merry ways.

I want you to know, though, that they did eventually change the sign. What a legacy.

STAYING THE COURSE

Many months into my chemo, Pauline, my oncologist, left for greener pastures far away, and there was a new sheriff in town for me. This was a great disappointment because I didn't see how Pauline could possibly be replaced. I liked her direct, no beating around the bush approach. She wasn't at all like that dastardly Dr. Pipe; Pauline had a unique way of delivering any bad news directly but with compassion, caring and love. Her skill set and deep, deep knowledge of her calling seemed to me beyond reproach. She wasn't everybody's cup of tea, as some couldn't handle the truth as well as others. I don't mean that as a criticism of some of the patients. It just means that people are different and some are more sensitive. That's just the way it is.

This is where I just know for absolute sure that God was looking after me. My new oncologist, Jim, was every bit as good as Pauline. His presence and relaxed attitude mirrored Pauline's and, like hers, didn't have that *I'm a doctor and you better know it* belligerence about it. He also had the added ingredient of, like me, having played rugby. Our warped sense of humor was matching, and we spent many a moment swapping jokes. He instructed everybody to call him Jim, even the staff members. All this may suggest he was a little loose and lackadaisical, which couldn't be further from the truth. When the moments were right, he was extremely attentive and applied his knowledge to whatever results came across his desk. He also continuously went on missions around the country, staying on top of the latest developments for treatments of the various cancers. He always stayed on the leading edge of his profession.

Part of my enjoyment with the group was when I could help them with my electrical knowledge. From time to time some of the group had electrical issues at home that were minor in complexity. I would drop by and fix the problem, which sometimes amounted to just re-setting a GFI. This was all part of the oneness we all felt toward each other. When I needed some support in other ways, physically or mentally, they were always there for me. For all of us, helping each other was a win-win situation. The love that flowed between all of us, like lava, helped us to relax and, at least for a short time, forget our woes.

It is well documented that fear and anxiety help feed the cancer and make it stronger. Was, y'know, the love thing a part of our cure? We shall never really know for sure, but I believed that we should use everything possible, including love, to attack the cancer that had invaded our bodies.

June, I believe, very subtly promoted this attitude during our meetings. As I have said before, she was a gem. I often thought there was an air of loving mystique watching over our domain. June, I know, had a large hand in that feeling of divine love that cloaked the whole area.

I think it is here that I want to share a story about where I took an enormous chance. About fifteen minutes into the group meeting one day, five people came through the front door. One was in a wheel chair, and the rest ambled in behind. We all said "Hi" and welcomed them all before continuing on in the normal fashion.

Our new member in the wheel chair explained, during her turn, that her whole immediate family was with her. She then proceeded to speak, for about fifteen minutes, about all of her woes. Her life, interrupted by multiple surgeries, had been a living nightmare over the last four months. Everyone was just dumbstruck by what this poor woman had endured, and the room had a huge black cloud dangling over it. When she finished, the area was in total silence.

This is where it gets dicey; I did a check with the spirit that I believe leads me before saying this and got the nod to go ahead, so I did. I said, "So, Gloria, other than that, is everything okay"? There wasn't even a moment's pause before everybody burst out laughing. The laughing went on forever with tears trickling down many a face. This included Gloria and her family members, who were in hysterics. The black cloud disappeared from whence it came, the dark side.

It seemed that my intuition was right to give me the green light, and I got away with a close one. During the post-session niceties, the newbies came over and thanked me for the humor and, like Ruth, said they knew they had come to the right place for comfort and support. I must admit saying that comment was risky. The last thing I wanted to do was alienate somebody from the get-go. They could have got the wrong idea about our sincerity and lost the chance of our support.

ALL WORK AND NO PLAY

Back at work it seemed that everybody had got used to my new lease on life. I had been breaking in a new young apprentice with the help of a wireman, Cory, I had already trained. One day, when the new apprentice had left and I was getting into the truck, Cory came over. He said the apprentice had told him he thought that I was an okay guy, but I had bad body odor that day.

I need to have an explanation here for those of you who may encounter this surgery. In nineteen years, a light gas release has happened to me only three times. This particular time, it was the result of having a really physically demanding day during the dog days of summer. I had been sweating profusely and drilling holes with a large drill, known as a "hole hog" all day. This caused a tiny gap between my skin and the adhesive holding the flange for the colostomy bag. Had I known, I could have just pressed on the flange to reattach it, and the problem wouldn't have occurred.

Anyway, Cory and I laughed about the situation, and the next day we talked to the newbie openly about everything over lunch. Yep, I know; such a delicate, lovely subject to discuss while eating. He couldn't believe that, (a) I had cancer and (b) I was working like I did while wearing the bag. He was embarrassed about what he'd said, but I put him at ease and we all had a little chuckle.

One bright and sunny early morning I turned left onto a one way road with blinker going and not a care in the world—that is, until a police car appeared behind me with Disney style lights flashing like crazy. I pulled over and rolled down the window. A large form blocked out the morning sun as a voice rumbled from the stomach and chest I was facing. A face did appear as the mountainous form bent down. "You didn't turn on your indicator when you turned," he said.

I told him that I jolly well had and distinctly remembered doing so. At that, he told me I wasn't wearing my seat belt. I wondered if he was going to go through a list until he found something I wasn't doing because I was wearing my seatbelt. Here is where it got funny. Because of my port, my chest was still very swollen and brightly colored, so I needed to put the shoulder strap under my armpit, which made the strap go lower across my body. As I explained this to the officer, I pulled down my T-shirt to show him my abstract painting. He jumped back, saying, "Oh my God that's…oh my God…carry on and have a nice day," his hand muffling his mouth.

Cory, who was with me, had seen my chest before and knew what the officer had seen. We both chuckled, no, laughed our heads off as we trundled on down the road. I often wonder if he put out a bulletin to all cars warning them not to pull me over.

Several weeks down the road my radiation treatments came to an end. I was still a very long way from finishing my chemo and continued to look forward to my week off every six weeks.

MY NEW PET

Another part of my new world was the introduction of positrom emission tomography, or PET scans. These tests were being conducted on a fairly regular basis so as to catch any recurrence of cancer quickly. On three separate occasions I was informed of some cancer possible in my lymph nodes in different parts of my body. While this was somewhat disconcerting it was good to know the medical staff was on top of things very quickly. I did feel relief from their prompt action and care.

Each time, these new areas of cancer needed to be eradicated from my body, of course. This required more minor operations and more anesthesia, which sent me into my other reality which I called La-La Land. It was a little disconcerting that the hospital staff knew my name without looking at their paper work. Hearing, "Oh, it's Barry. Just wheel him into room seven," seemed a little odd. One day I imagined I saw a room with my name on it in gold letters.

My body was starting to look like it had been thrown off a three hundred foot cliff. My scar count was going up by the month as they kept removing those imposing cancerous lymph nodes. It began to seem like we were chasing those pesky things around my body, rather like those games at the fairground—you know, where you hit a rat head that pops up and them another pops up and you hit that and so forth.

Each time something was found it meant more and more PET scans, of course. Would they never end? I was sure they would because I was going to beat this thing if it killed me. (I thought that was funny even if nobody else did.) I recall something funny Mark Twain once said. He was walking down the road with a friend in torrential rain. The rain had been incessant for four days and the friend asked, "Is it ever going to stop raining"? Mark Twain replied, "It always has." So I was thinking the same thing: *This too shall pass.*

The PET scans were, as was usual for me, done as the first patient in the morning. A traveling truck unit came to the hospital on Tuesdays and did their thing. Again, I got to know everybody really well, and I obviously also got to know the routine. I would go into a small room at one end of the truck and get comfortable in a relaxing recliner. After the weight, height, blood pressure and temperature details were taken, I would be injected with radioactive isotopes. They would dim the lights and leave for half an hour or so before taking me to the PET scan machine. If I wanted to read, I just used the glow emanating from my body. I'm joking, but I would sometimes wonder about that.

Stripped to almost nothing, I would have to lay prone on a sliver of a table with my knees raised before being slid into the chamber automatically. They did place a cushioned, curved contraption under my knees for comfort. I also had a nice warm blanket covering my vulnerable body. I needed to remain as still as possible for about forty minutes, if I remember correctly. The auto table would move me back and forth slightly at various times with all kinds of noises and whirring going on simultaneously.

To relax myself I would sing that HU song to myself. It really helped me to remain calm and stationary. The crew would always comment on how great the images were and were impressed by my tenacity in keeping still. When I told them my secret, they were intrigued enough to ask many questions about my spirituality. Unlike the one doctor, they believed that positive thinking and religion could help in the cure of disease.

One morning when I went for a scan they couldn't get the PET machine to start up. I was all wired up and needled to take the juice and was asked if I minded waiting for a while. Of course I was cool with that but wondered what was up. After an hour or so they told me I couldn't get tested that day as the isotopes had a very short half-life and were not reliable enough now after the wait. Oh well, I would have to wait until the following Tuesday.

When I arrived the next week my first question was, "So what happened last week?" It turns out it had been very simple to fix. The machine wouldn't start because the truck wasn't perfectly level. They could have leveled the truck via the four hydraulic motors on each corner, but no alarms told them it was out of kilter, and they didn't think of that resolution. They profusely apologized up hill and down dale, but it wasn't necessary. The world was still turning at the same speed, so no harm done.

My lifestyle change regime was staying on track and balanced. I had weekly chemo on Monday, was buggered by Thursday, rested up on Saturday and Sunday, recouped by Monday, and then it was *Play it again, Sam*. One problem was that the chemo was getting harder and harder to administer to me, and nobody knew why. The staff was a little flummoxed and tried all kinds of remedies but to no avail. I helped some by raising my arm above my head and pulling my left shoulder backwards. They did express their gratitude for me not whining and complaining.

THE FIRST END GAME AND THEN

Fifteen months later, completing my chemo was a huge milestone. I was clear of cancer and life was good. Going to work was still tiring for a while but was getting better and better.

My doctors' visits and PET scans continued, and the support group was still going strong. Some of the members warned me about saying I was clear of cancer, y'know, *cured*. They said I was in remission, not cured. I looked up the word remission and it means something like, "We think the cancer is gone, but we're not sure so give it some time." My take on this was "If the tests showed no cancer and the docs verify that, then I don't have cancer."

"What if it comes back?" said the pessimists. To which I said, "Then I would have cancer again, but right now I do not have cancer." This back and forth continued for weeks with most members buying into my argument, especially Ruth. It became a popular standing conversation with a lot of jovial comments between us.

My next spiritual move may shock some of you readers. After a couple of weeks, I went into contemplation before going to sleep, as was quite normal for me. I was deep into another world when I asked my spiritual leader a unique question. I said, "If and only if I have any more karma to work off regarding cancer, I am prepared to do it now. If not, then let it be and don't take any action." I knew I was strong enough mentally and physically, and I had a wonderful support group around me. I had a fantastic wife who would be by my side no matter what, with love. I had a great work boss who would stand by me, along with a super hospital staff and organization and many good friends. I was willing to finish the karma if need be.

Two weeks later I got my answer.

I'd had yet another glow in the dark PET scan. This was nothing out of the ordinary for me. Two days later, Laraine and I went to see Jim, the oncologist, for the results. We were ushered into an exam room as usual, but something wasn't right. Have you ever had that feeling that somebody is behind you and it makes you turn around? There was an air of that kind of uneasiness, and it seemed more quiet than normal. The staff was friendly but the smiling was different somehow. Anyway, we sat down and the first person in the room was June. This was unusual; she had never been in the room before when I was getting results or a checkup. Maybe she just wanted to see me? Next into the room came Jim, who closed the door, as doctors do. He smiled while shaking my hand but looked more serious than normal. My regular statistics had already been taken and were fine, so why the glum face?

"Barry," he said, "especially for somebody like you, I hate to report that your cancer has come back." June put her hand on mine as she sat just to the side of Laraine and me. My head dropped along with my heart as tears welled in my eyes. Laraine squeezed my other hand and had tears in her eyes as Jim looked on with sadness and a frown upon his face.

Silence was the order of the day as June and Jim let the news sink in. This was so classy of them. When they could see we were calming down and over the initial shock, Jim spoke again. He told us that the colon cancer was in my spine. You see, as I had learned over the past year, cancer is not just cancer. Different types of cancer can move to other parts of the body and still be called, for instance, colon cancer.

June then expressed her thought that we could beat this dreaded disease just like before. My/our attitude, along with treatment, could overcome this wrenching setback. I knew that I had been chasing the cancer around my lymph system with great success for a while but thought I was out of the woods. She encouraged me not to give up, to keep going.

GETTING RADICAL

The panel of oncologists would discuss my latest results and come up with a plan at their weekly meeting. I did like this approach. All the brains of the cancer center would give all their different opinions, and a resulting treatment would ensue.

The powers that be decided that they want me to undergo 44 more treatments of radiation. My body was already glowing from radiation and multiple MRI and PET scans; move over Chernobyl, there's a new sheriff in town. The good news was that they determined I was not going to have to have more chemo, at least not until they saw if the radiation nailed it.

We went over to the radiation side of the cancer center to organize my next step. That was all I could focus on at that moment in time. The radiologist went through all the films again and explained all the details and plans for the next round of treatments.

He showed where in four of my vertebrae the cancer had struck. There were bore holes going through the bone like Swiss cheese. It was as if worms had been boring away, as in a bad apple. It was quite a shocker for me to look at and absorb the severity of the situation. I imagined being paralyzed from the waist down because of cancer eating through my spinal column, but I tried to dismiss the fear. I tried to remember *Always look to the light and the positive side of life.* That was easier said than done.

From the radiation center, I was invited to a prep room where I was to be exposed again for four more tattoos. Throughout my fifteen year Royal Navy career, I had fought off the temptation to get tattoos. Now I was the proud owner of eight of them. Unless I am on a nude beach, though, those eight little crosses don't show.

I was to start the radiation the following week, which was only three days away. Again, I set the procedures up for the first of the day so I could get to work on time. They warned me that I might not be able to handle working this second time around, but my mind didn't even listen to that kind of negativity. I knew they were just thinking of my welfare and basing their warning on previous experiences with patients. My own positive belief system had to take the forefront of this scenario.

At my first zapping I lay prostrate once more before what I thought of as the radiation death ray machine while they lined it up with my crosses. The crew welcomed me back while wishing they didn't have to. At least we could continue swapping jokes.

Twenty minutes later I was on my way, feeling none the worse for wear.

I was going to be working by myself about ten miles southwest of town out in the country. There was a new development of about 140 houses, and I had wired maybe a dozen or so of them. The new owners of one of the homes, after about six months, had decided to finish their basement. They knew me from many meetings I'd had with them about customizing their electrical requirements. I was to be their man for the job.

After an hour had passed, I started to feel nauseous and swallowed deeply several times. This happened two more times before I dashed outside to the garden. I made it outside before unloading breakfast along with any other particles that wanted to participate. After depositing my stomach contents to fertilize the plants, I felt a lot better and returned to the job at hand.

It wasn't ten minutes later that the whole scene started over. This time I did remember there was a bathroom in the basement. I barely made it to the bowl before regurgitating more than I thought was still inside of me. Again, I felt a lot better for unloading my storage locker, so after a few minutes got back to work. Five minutes later I was back in trouble. If I'd been pregnant, it would be like my contractions were getting closer and closer.

I was now feeling very weak and decided to head for the cancer center. I slowly made it up the stairs and explained to the homeowner what was going on before heading for the truck. I was only two miles down the road when I had to pull over and, without success, tried to heave my stomach into my mouth. I was now weaker than before and fading fast. Twice more before hitting the edge of town I lunged for the grass as my now dry heaves were causing great pain and were extremely acidic.

Still three miles or so from the cancer center, I pulled over on a fairly busy street and lay on the ground to heave. I was so weak I could not get back up and into the truck, so I stayed on the ground. I hoped that a passing car would stop and assist or at least call 911, but this did not happen. What happened to my friendly town of helpful people? They probably thought I was some drunk from the night before who made it back to work. Even now, I can't understand why I was left to rot in the gutter. One hears of all these good Samaritans helping people all the time, but that wasn't the case for me, not that day. I did eventually get up the strength to climb back into the high cab and get closer to my goal, the cancer center.

My next stop was, in fact, outside the cancer center doors. I did not park the truck in a designated spot but got as close to the entry doors as possible. I literally crawled on the ground toward the automatic doors and made it through the first set. As I progressed forward the second set of doors slid open. The two receptionists looked up and I think, just for a second, thought

I was messing with them. I earned that because I was always pulling some kind of prank on them and having a whale of a time. They must have seen the desperate, anguished look on my face and leapt into action, calling for help and grabbing a wheelchair.

Five people were soon around me holding the chair, lifting me, and doing everything possible in a wonderfully coordinated dance. I was whisked into the area where I had received chemo, and an IV was into my port quicker than you can say Jack Robinson.

Jim, the oncologist, was by my side in nothing flat and authorized the induction of saline into my body. I was fussed over continuously until I got my faculties back. I noticed many a tear by the staff, especially the registration ladies. They were, more than likely, not as used to such traumatic incidents as the rest of the staff.

I was ordered to stay for the rest of the day for observation and lots more saline. John, my boss, was called and he came to pick up the truck. He was very concerned and stayed for a short while as a good friend would. Laraine came to the center as quick as she could and stayed until I could go home.

Before leaving, I was taken to the radiology department, where I had a consultation. Their take on this incident was that I was considered to be very strong, and they had thought I could deal with the high dose of radiation they gave me for the first session. This was based on how I had handled it during my earlier course of treatments. However, they overdid it a tad. They reduced the dosage but then had to increase the amount of times I got zapped. The amount of radiation was to be the same, ergo, lower dosage equaled more treatments.

Much to Laraine's chagrin, I did go to work the next day. John was a little skeptical as well and made sure I had an apprentice with me this time. The home owner whose basement I was wiring was also very concerned for me, which was nice. Looking back, I am sorry I put Laraine through the worry she must have suffered all day long. But I needed to work; remember, that was my lifeline to survival and being cured. I was determined to punch through the barricade of fire and brimstone I was going through.

FACING THE SUPPORT GROUP

The next cancer support meeting was interesting. When it came to my turn to talk, I said, "Pass," so they knew something was up. June kept an eye on me, and I signaled her when I was ready to give the bad news. Naturally, she knew all of what was happening. She had come into the infusion room while I was being hydrated to talk to me about how I felt and give me her full support. June was and always will be an angel in my eyes. She always had the right balance of what to do and say.

    I broke down a little as I told them the news. Of course everybody was very sad for me, but I tried not to let them get too down about it. The naysayers who had warned me of my, to them, misguided optimism were in full voice, though. I repeated my mantra: I had been clear of cancer. Now I merely had cancer again." I vowed to fight it again just as before. Yes, it did concern me more. What if it came back again? And what about again and again? I dashed those thoughts from my mind as I could only deal with what I had, not what I might someday have. It would be like me inviting it to stay for good, rather than a short visit.

With a radiation level now acceptable to my body, life went on. In this second round, I did get so very tired during the pounding of my bodily resources, but as before I was determined to soldier on, regardless. Working daily was still my lifeline for survival.

Luckily, the ship righted. Eight weeks later, I received the great news that the radiation had done the trick. My cancer was gone again.

I am a firm believer in doing everything you can at all times. Some people just want to try one thing at a time, and that's their choice. But I would rather sling any kind of mud at the wall—no matter if it's medical, physical, mental, or spiritual—just like my friend Ruth had done for herself. If it sticks, great, if it doesn't, so what? I tried.

Some members of the support group again warned me about saying I was cured. I gave them the same answer I'd given before: "If it comes back, I have cancer again. Right now all the tests show I have no cancer." My believers cheered, of course, and the others booed. It was all in fun, and we moved on with everybody laughing and smiling.

It wasn't long after finding out about my second cancer career that David got the same news I had earlier; his cancer had returned. He was, as could be expected, devastated. He was beside himself and in great pain physically and emotionally. His bemoaning attitude was easily understood by most but not all in our group. Some took the attitude that he needed to pull up his socks. They didn't say that, but that is the impression they gave.

He told the group that he was going to refuse treatment and go home to his mother and quietly pass away. The Fab Four had a long talk with him after the meeting and told him that we supported him. We respected his choice because we knew the hardships he had suffered with his treatment. His body hadn't handled it the way mine had. Also, his journey had been more painful from the outset. Because he was uninsured, he couldn't have a port inserted, and he couldn't have his treatment administered at the cancer center. He was a very nice and respectable person who had been plunged into depression through no fault of his own. I thought, overall, he was very strong and brave.

At the next support group meeting, after I brought up the subject, we spoke about our role as a support group, not a judgment group. However a person wanted to handle their situation, we should be there to support them. Any other role would be handled by June and various doctors.

David did leave us a few weeks later, passing away peacefully surrounded by loved ones.

DEPARTING IS SUCH SWEET SORROW

Mavis, our marijuana puffing friend who was now totally accepted by almost everybody, decided to throw a party at her house for the group. Dave, her husband, was fully on board and instrumental in putting it all together. It was a glorious sunny Saturday afternoon with clear mountains and a crystal clear blue sky. Mavis was in full cry with her strong Irish accent, cigarette in mouth and a bottle of beer in her hand. She was full of life, visiting with all and sundry while cheering them all up. The party got louder and more raucous as the afternoon marched on.

As people gradually slipped away, I wanted to be one of the last to leave. I knew, or at least I thought I knew, that all was not as rosy as it appeared. As Mavis, Dave, Laraine and I started to clear the area of the aftermath of plates and cups, I maneuvered alongside Mavis and whispered, "This is about your last hurrah isn't it?"

She replied, "Yeah. Well, nothing like going out with a bang and attending my own wake." We both sat down as I held her hand. My eyes were wet as I held back my tears. Her love and grace during her retreat from this world was a thing of beauty. We smiled at each other and stayed silent for a while. I proceeded to tell her of the joy and frankness she always brought to the group. Her infectious laugh was certainly going to be missed. She asked me not to divulge her situation, and I honored that. Mavis did attend one more meeting a couple of weeks later, and then it was time for her to leave.

Her Catholic funeral was well attended with easily over one hundred people at the church. It was my first Catholic funeral in perhaps forty years, and I remember the priest holding this urn type thing on a chain and swinging it from side to side with smoke (incense, I believe) pouring out of it. I thought of dousing him with a nearby fire extinguisher. I'm just kidding, but I needed to lighten up a little. The food afterwards was magnificent with a layout like a banquet at Buckingham Palace. Mavis's zest for fun and life was apparent throughout this festive time, and we all enjoyed moments of reflection. We all missed her vitality and frivolity.

At the next support group meeting, the candle we burned for Mavis seemed to be doing a jig. The flame was light and bright and full of life, just like her. I stared at it in a trance-like state and let my imagination take over. I saw Mavis in that light and watched her dance with an Irish fling added into the mix. I was a million miles away with a smile on my face before snapping back to reality as June blew my fantasy flame out. It was time to say goodbye.

This parting of ways was repeated on too many occasions, and yet the number of survivors was quite extraordinary. Our center's successes far outweighed our losses. We enjoyed each other's company, and life, while somewhat arduous at times, was good. The support group really worked for the benefit of all.

LETTING GO AND A CLOSE CALL

The chemo was finished for sure, and radiation was in the history books. Jim, the oncologist, wanted to wait a year or more before removing the port in my chest. It wasn't a nuisance and we were still at the stage of "What if?" My checkups were now three months apart, and the PET scans were every six months.

All was going well. Then one day Jim said he didn't need to see me again for six months instead of three, and there was no need for another PET scan. One would think this would have been a joyous moment, but it had an adverse effect on me. How would I know if the cancer came back? My backup system was gone; so was my confidence in always being clear of cancer. This was a worry I hadn't foreseen.

My mind was a mess for quite a while, and not having PET scans took some getting used to. I did eventually stop worrying about it, but it took a long time, a long time.

Although I had no more PET scans or chemo, I did go to the Cancer Center every six weeks to have the port and its tube cleaned out. As always, I arranged to go first thing in the morning so I could get to work. They would flush saline into and out of the mechanism. I bring this up because each time we did this, it got harder and harder to shoot in the saline. Finally, the nurses told me they wanted to have me get an X-ray to see what was going on. I told them not to bother. I could handle it. They insisted, and after several back and forth exchanges, they called in the doctor.

Of course the doctor immediately took the nurses' side, and off I went to X-ray. I was stretched out with a monitor screen just to the right of my head for me to see inside myself, showing everything as in a window. I set the place alight as it revealed that the tube from the disc in my chest to the artery had broken off. This six inch tube was inside my heart and diagonally across it through a valve. Bodies flew everywhere, and I heard somebody say, "Quick, get Doctor Joiner." I asked what was going on, and they said I was going straight into surgery to remove the tube.

This seemed a trifle worrying to me, and I wondered if I could get to work later that day; I was busy, you know. I then heard a nurse say that we were lucky; they had caught the surgeon getting into his car to go home. Apparently he had just finished an early morning surgery and was leaving the hospital.

They were about to start prepping me with needles and such to put me out for the count. So I asked to borrow a phone. I needed to let John, my boss, know and also to update my wife. I didn't want to panic Laraine, so I coolly asked her if she could come to the hospital to drive me home as I had been given a drug that made it dangerous to drive. Within seconds I was onto another gurney and being whisked down a hallway to an operating room. The surgeon was scooting the other way, still with his civilian clothes on. We said "hi" to each other with a smile.

I was only three quarters unconscious as they needed me to move during a part of the procedure. I lay prone, feeling loosey-goosey as I counted the tiles in the ceiling. In came the corps of engineers, and off to the races we went. In my three-quarter stupor I started to tell some jokes. Since I was somewhat out of it, some of them were rather rugged. I spoke softly, so I kept having to repeat them as the team exchanged places. The place was in virtual uproar until the surgeon said I had to stop. He was starting to laugh and he had this grabber arm up my artery near the heart. It was getting dangerous.

The next thing I knew, I was in a hospital room waking up to a nurse and Laraine looking at me and smiling. Laraine was holding my hand, an all too familiar task for her over the last couple of years.

The hospital staff handed me the tube they pulled out and, sure enough, it was just over six inches long. I still have it somewhere in the house. A day later I was at home; I returned to work the following Monday.

A few weeks later I got a $1000.00 bill from the hospital—my 20% share of the cost of the procedure. I felt I shouldn't have to pay this as I had found out the tube was run between my collar bone and top rib. Eventually the chafing had cut the tube and it had flowed into my heart. I mean, jiminy, it could have killed me. The powers that be insisted I pay, even after multiple phone arguments, and I looked doomed to oblige.

When talking this over with June, she said she would set up a meeting with a person from a kind of hospital damage control committee. She also told me she would accompany me to the meeting and just listen.

Two days later, before a support group meeting, I sat with June and the damage control lady. I felt bad about complaining because this hospital had been wonderful to me and had saved my life on more than one occasion. Still, the problem had not been my fault. The surgery was the fault of the tube from the port being placed in a poor position, I explained. Therefore, I shouldn't have to pay. I also pointed out that $1000.00 was a drop in the bucket for them but not for me. I followed that up with, "Surely, court costs would be more than that, and I can't see a jury siding with the hospital." This was a last resort and I felt bad about it.

The damage control lady stood firm, but as we parted ways she told me she would bring it up at the next committee meeting and call me with the result. I thought, "Fair enough," and carried on to the support group meeting with June. I asked her what she thought of what I had said, and she told me I had said all the right things. She also said I shouldn't feel bad; it was what they dealt with all the time.

First thing the next morning, I got I call from the damage control woman. My bill for $1000.00 had been rescinded. Since there had been no time for a committee meeting, I believe she had made up her mind up the previous evening.

At my doctor's request, a new port was put in for free, free to me anyway. His reasoning was that if my cancer did come back, everything would be ready. I had been chasing the lymph node system around trying to completely eradicate the cancer, and he needed to be sure of it not returning for a little longer. Cancer was always lying in wait at the back of my mind.

As time went on checkup times stretched to a year apart, and after five years they fell away completely. Again a strange feeling came over me. I was happy but somewhat apprehensive. Five years is a long time to have a port in one's chest.

MOVING DAY

Christmases came and went, and a new life was approaching. The handwriting was on the wall regarding my current job. I knew the office manager they had hired a year or so earlier had been lying about me and had been changing my paperwork to make me look bad. I was written up for some really stupid little thing. It was one of those, "So what would you have done differently under the circumstances I was faced with?" incidents. Then I was written up again for not reporting a very minor injury in a timely manner. I did have the forms filled out, but I was getting to the office in the morning before anybody was there and leaving before anybody had unlocked it, and getting back to the office after everybody was gone. I would have normally unlocked and gone in, but my key had been taken away a month earlier. Hmmmm, clue after clue, but I had given so much to that company and respected both owners so much, I didn't want to leave. There was nothing I could do, so trusted in the gods that this was meant to be.

Of course, eventually, the day of reckoning came and it was time to go. John called me into the office on that fateful Monday morning, and I knew why. He was looking very sad and even had a few tears. John was a big man and looked the part of a strapping, strong boss, and he was. While we had a great relationship, the manager had gotten to his wife enough that she had no alternative but to insist I was let go. That was my take, anyway. I have no hard feelings and have always wished them well; they were very good to me and I will always be so grateful.

I was unemployed for less than a day when I got a phone call from another company. The jungle drums travel far and fast. I was asked if I would like to help out an electrical contractor who had a bubble of work and needed help. We met, and he explained it would be just until he got through this busy time. He suggested that I use this time to find a good job and if one came up, to leave him and take it. This way he was helping himself and helping me. Wow. I had fallen into you know what and come up smelling like roses.

Six months later he drove up to a job site one day and apologetically told me it was time to leave. He was caught up and, actually, had been for quite a while but kept me on as long as he could. I told him off, tongue in cheek. He had done me a great service and apologies were out of the question. He was a very nice person and upright and honest.

Two days later I was employed by a company where I quickly decided I fit like a square peg in a round hole. I was grateful for their willingness to hire me, and they were good people, but they were quite the rednecks. The main conversations were about guns and trucks and the like. Fortunately, another company was soon hired to do half the work that this company did, and I was let go. I understood—last in, first out. One laid off employee had worked for them for twelve years.

I knew this layoff would eventually work out to be in my best interest; I just wasn't sure how yet. I needed to trust in God's plan and not my own. Many religions teach this approach, and so does my spiritual path. When I look back into my personal history, all of my seemingly bad situations have always turned out for the best.

I spent the next two weeks doing work for contractor friends—you know, smaller jobs that the big boys generally didn't want. I was then interviewed for a permanent job with a fairly new startup company. The owner didn't want to pay me what I was worth but really wanted me. Instead, he ended up hiring an inferior journeyman who lasted two weeks. I was interviewed again, but it was more or less for him to try and talk me into less pay. I was not greedy and was asking less than a very experienced journeyman would normally get. I was not going to give my hard work and loyalty away for less than it was worth.

One week later I got a call from The Home Depot, where I had also been interviewed, and was hired. They wanted a tradesman with master electrician status in every store, and I fit the bill. They would pay me the same wages as my last employer. This was actually a $300 a month pay raise as my insurance was that much less at The Home Depot while actually being better. They also gave bonuses and other monetary rewards if they were earned. I found these rewards easy to earn as all I had to do was my job.

I was inside in the cold of the winter and heat of the summer—what a joy. I got to train home owners and help contractors. They would discuss jobs with me and I could get them the right equipment quickly and also remind them of items they might have forgotten on their list. Was this a great life or what?

The hours I had to work made it difficult for me to attend the cancer support group. I did drop in rather late into a session from time to time, but for the most part it was the end. I had been going for around six years at this juncture, so maybe it was just my time to leave the group.

HELP IS ON THE WAY

My feet were well and truly under the table at The Home Depot, an excellent company to work for, by the way. But a new element was coming into my life.

One day a regular customer came in and told me a member of his family had just been diagnosed with cancer. He knew of my earlier diagnosis and spilled his heart out to me. I spoke with him for well over half an hour and had one eye on my supervisor, worried about the amount of time I was spending with one customer.

Still, I helped the customer feel much more at ease with the news and said to him, with a huge smile on my face, "Hey, look at me. I am fine. Cancer is no longer a certain death sentence." He left much better off than when he had come in.

After the long time spent with said customer, I went to my supervisor to apologize and explain why. His response surprised me; he told me it was perfectly okay. The Home Depot encourages bonding with the customers and making personal connections. It's good for business.

I wondered, *Have the gods put me here to not only assist regular customers but to be a support for people concerned about cancer?*

Maybe so. Throughout my tenure at The Home Depot, which took me to retirement, I helped many people, several of whom were employees. One person even came in to ask if I would facilitate her husband's memorial service, to which I agreed. She knew I was a cleric for my spiritual path of Eckankar and trusted me. She also knew her husband and I had had many conversations during his battle with cancer.

I facilitated another memorial service for an employee whose wife had succumbed to this awful disease. We had become great friends, and I even visited the hospital with him during the last few weeks of her life. He was feeling alone and, I am sure, scared. It was touching to see him gently and slowly brush her hair, love in his eyes. Mostly she was either asleep or in a comatose state and you could see his love for her. I mostly didn't say anything, but I was a physical and mental support for him and I felt grateful and honored to be there for him.

LIFE IS GOOD

I have lived for nineteen years with my friend, the colostomy. The people in DVDs about life with colostomy bags try to tell you how normal everything will be for you. Some even say how they wouldn't want to go back to being normal, bowel-wise. I find that hard to swallow. I am not one of those people and would jump at the chance to reverse my state.

That being said, I am at ease with the situation and am very grateful for this alternative. I am also very grateful for being given the opportunity to help so many people. Many people have cancer, know a friend with cancer, or have a family member going through cancer. If I can help them all in some small way, then it was worth getting the cancer myself. I know, it sounds crazy doesn't it?

I continue to speak freely about cancer to anybody who needs to hear. It's amazing how often a person needs some reassurance or just an ear to speak to. It gets easier and easier to help more and more people. Yes, the joy I get from having had cancer is enormous, but I still don't recommend it as a deliberate side job.

ADVICE FOR CANCER PATIENTS AND CARE GIVERS

My friend in Florida has a saying: *This is your train Jesse, you rob it any way you want.* I have a few suggestions for cancer patients and caretakers, but remember: You are the captain of your ship. Steer her well. Good luck.

- Let your feelings out
- Let your feelings in. In other words, allow yourself to feel what you feel.
- Only share when you are ready.
- Only share when *they,* meaning loved ones, are ready.
- Don't be afraid to cry.
- When ready, let people in and accept their help.
- Don't be afraid; you can worry though.
- Caregivers, give plenty of space.
- Caregivers, remember that you have feelings, too. And that's okay.
- Protect each other but don't go overboard.
- Allow others to do what they think is best for you spiritually or religiously because it helps *them.* You

can always ignore or reject what they say silently to yourself
- Do everything you can do. It helps, if possible, to keep moving.
- Only give up when there is no more to do. If times improve, try to help others.
- Make time for yourself.
- Keep your friends.
- Dump your enemies.
- Keep your chin up.

If cancer does cross your path, grab it, own it and fight it in every way possible to you at the time. Don't get angry at it, don't let it win, and most of all, kick butt!

May the blessings be to you all.

ABOUT THE AUTHOR

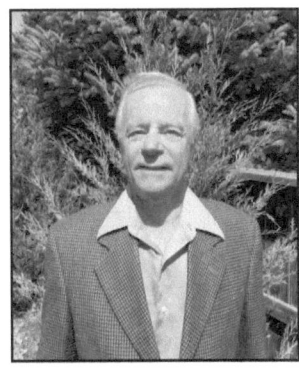

Barry "Jack" Frost has been a cancer survivor for 19 years. He grew up in Lewes, England, traveled the world with the Royal Navy for 15 years, then married an American and moved to the United States. Before retirement, he worked as an electrical specialist, using skills he learned in his years with the Navy for many organizations, including a company that built communication systems for the Space Shuttle.

He is also the author of *Life in a Blue Suit—A Sailor's Tales of Grit, Humor, Loyalty, and Leadership in the Royal Navy.*

You can contact Frost at sirbfrost@msn.com.

Made in United States
Troutdale, OR
04/12/2024